EASY TO PREPARE DIVERTICULITIS

DIET COOKBOOK

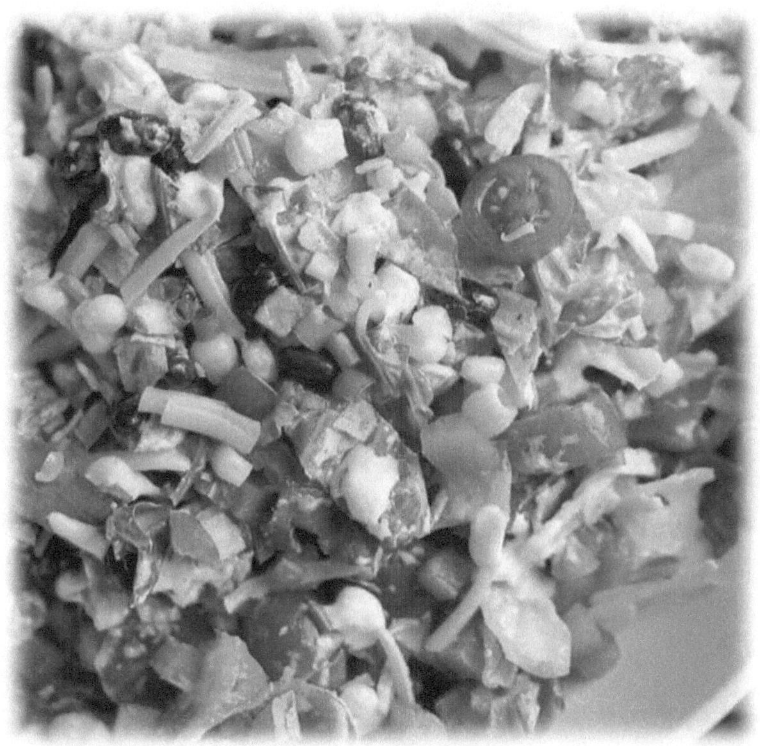

Low Fiber Meals to Soothe Inflammation and

Prevent Painful Flare-Ups

LAKEISHA OWENS

TABLE OF CONTENT

INTRODUCTION

"EASY TO PREPARE DIVERTICULITIS DIET COOKBOOK" serves as an invaluable resource for individuals navigating the complexities of diverticulitis, a condition characterized by the formation of diverticula in the digestive tract which can lead to painful inflammation or infection. This book is structured to cater to the needs of those who are newly diagnosed with diverticulitis, as well as those looking to maintain their health after recovery from an acute episode. Central to the " EASY TO PREPARE DIVERTICULITIS DIET COOKBOOK" is its extensive collection of recipes specifically tailored to be gentle on the digestive system while being nutritious and satisfying. Each recipe within the cookbook is crafted with the dual goals of minimizing the risk of diverticulitis flare-ups and promoting overall digestive health. Ingredients are carefully selected to avoid those that are known to aggravate the condition, such as seeds, nuts, and certain fibrous foods, especially in the early stages. Instead, the focus is on whole, nutrient-dense foods that support healing and well-being.

When managing diverticulitis, especially during a flare-up, it's crucial to follow a diet that minimizes irritation to the digestive system. During the acute phase, a clear liquid or very low fiber diet may be recommended by your healthcare provider, gradually transitioning to more solid foods as inflammation decreases.

HAPPY COOKING!!!!!!!!

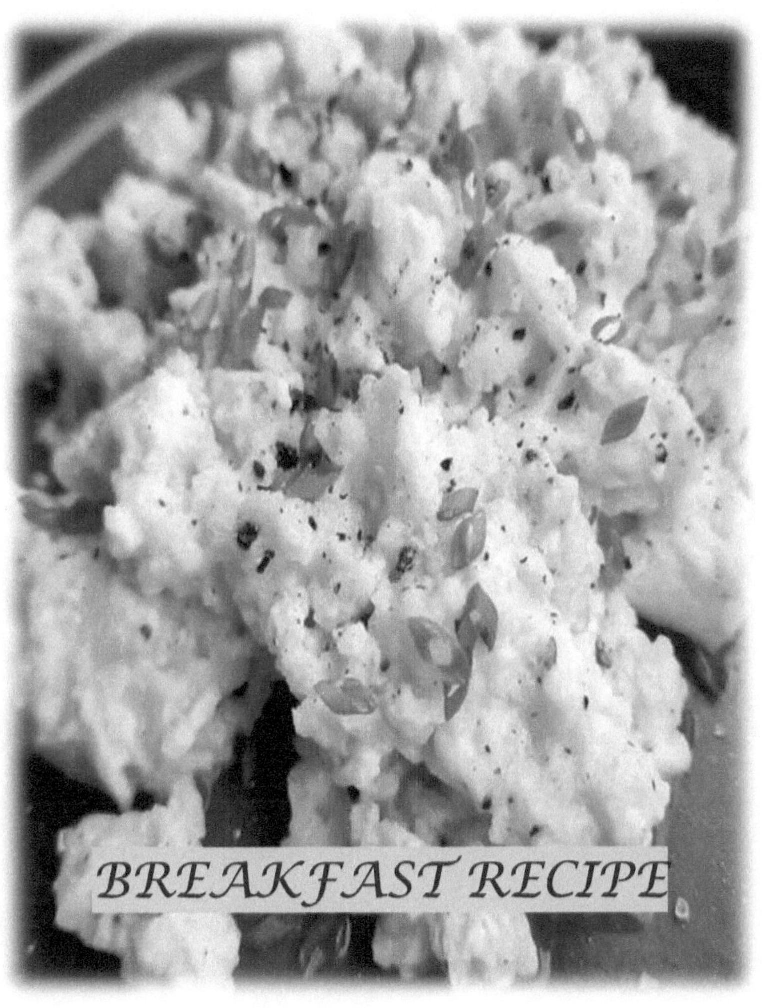

BREAKFAST RECIPE

The following breakfast recipes are designed with a focus on being gentle on the digestive system.

RECIPES

BREAKFAST RECIPE

Smooth Scrambled Eggs

Ingredients:

2 large eggs

2 tablespoons milk

Salt to taste

1 tablespoon unsalted butter

Instructions:

Whisk the eggs, milk, and a pinch of salt together until smooth.

Melt butter in a non-stick pan over low heat.

Add the egg mixture, and gently stir until softly set.

Low-Fiber French Toast

Ingredients:

2 slices white bread (low fiber)

1 egg

1/4 cup milk

1/2 teaspoon vanilla extract

Butter for frying

Maple syrup (for serving)

Instructions:

Whisk together egg, milk, and vanilla in a shallow dish.

Soak bread slices in the mixture for 1 minute each side.

Melt butter in a skillet over medium heat.

Cook bread until golden brown on both sides.

Serve with a drizzle of maple syrup.

Creamy Polenta

Ingredients:

1/2 cup polenta (cornmeal)

2 cups water

1/4 teaspoon salt

1 tablespoon butter

1/4 cup grated Parmesan cheese.

Instructions:

Bring water and salt to a boil in a saucepan.

Gradually whisk in the polenta.

Reduce heat to low and cook, stirring frequently, until creamy and thick, about 20 minutes.

Stir in butter and Parmesan cheese until well combined.

Baked Custard

Ingredients:

2 large eggs

2 cups milk

1/4 cup sugar

1/2 teaspoon vanilla extract

Nutmeg (optional)

Instructions:

Preheat oven to 325°F (165°C).

Whisk eggs, milk, sugar, and vanilla together until smooth.

Pour into ramekins.

Sprinkle with nutmeg if desired.

Place ramekins in a baking dish and fill the dish with boiling water halfway up the sides of the ramekins.

Bake for 45 minutes or until set.

Simple Oat Porridge

Ingredients:

1/2 cup rolled oats (choose quick-cooking for lower fiber)

1 cup water or milk

Pinch of salt

Instructions:

Combine oats, water/milk, and salt in a saucepan.

Bring to a boil, then reduce heat to simmer, stirring frequently, until desired consistency is reached.

Soft Poached Egg on White Toast

Ingredients:

1 large egg

1 slice white bread (low-fiber)

Butter

Instructions:

Poach the egg gently in simmering water until the whites are set but the yolk is still runny.

Toast the bread and spread with butter.

Place the poached egg on the toast and season with salt to taste.

Rice Porridge (Congee)

Ingredients:

1/2 cup white rice

4 cups water

Pinch of salt

Instructions:

Rinse the rice until the water runs clear.

Combine rice, water, and salt in a pot and bring to a boil.

Reduce heat to a simmer, cover, and cook, stirring occasionally, until the rice is very soft and the mixture is creamy, about 1 hour.

Mashed Potato Pancakes

Ingredients:

1 cup mashed potatoes

1 egg, beaten

2 tablespoons flour

Salt to taste

Butter for frying

Instructions:

Mix mashed potatoes, egg, flour, and salt in a bowl.

Heat butter in a skillet over medium heat.

Drop spoonfuls of the mixture into the skillet, flatten, and fry

until golden brown on both sides.

Cream of Wheat

Ingredients:

1/4 cup cream of wheat (farina)

1 cup water or milk

Pinch of salt

Instructions:

Bring water or milk to a boil in a saucepan.

Gradually whisk in the cream of wheat and salt.

Reduce heat to low and cook, stirring constantly, until thickened, about 2-3 minutes.

Remember, during a diverticulitis flare-up, it's essential to start with a liquid or very low fiber diet and gradually reintroduce solid foods as recommended by your healthcare provider. These recipes should be adapted to your current dietary phase and tolerance.

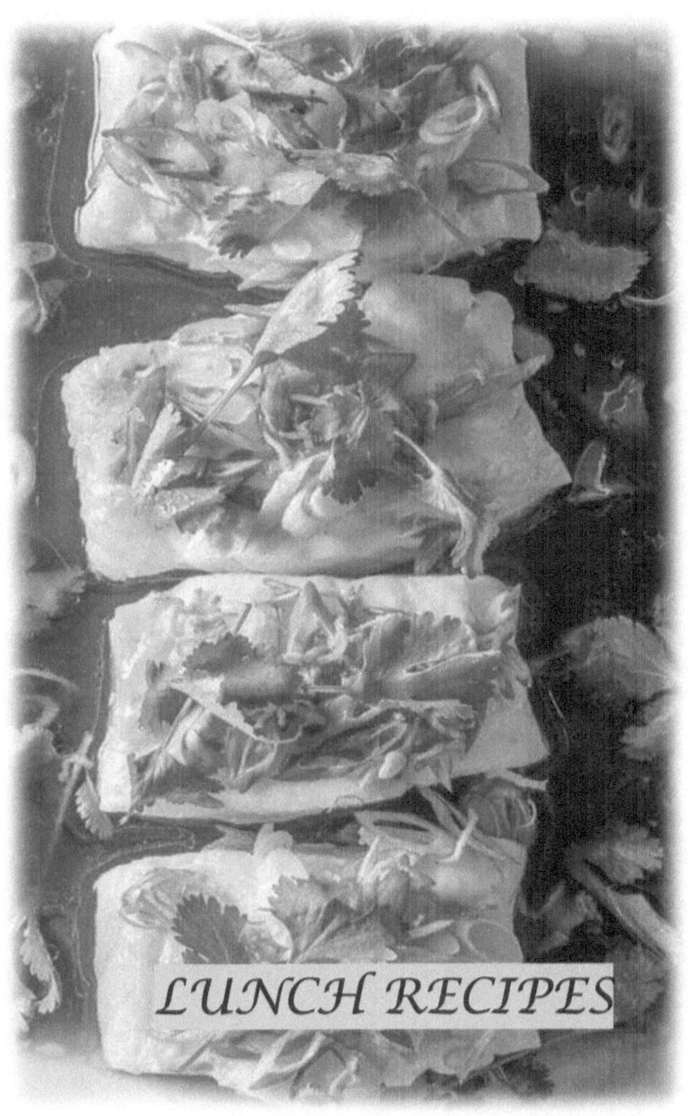
LUNCH RECIPES

Creating lunch recipes for those with diverticulitis involves focusing on meals that are gentle on the digestive system, particularly during a flare-up.

Chicken and Rice Soup

Ingredients:

2 cups low-sodium chicken broth

1/2 cup cooked white rice

1/2 cup cooked, shredded chicken breast

Salt and pepper to taste

Instructions:

In a pot, bring the chicken broth to a simmer.

Add the cooked rice and shredded chicken to the pot.

Season with salt and pepper, and simmer for 10-15 minutes until heated through.

Baked White Fish with Herbs

Ingredients:

2 white fish fillets (such as tilapia or cod)

1 tablespoon olive oil

1 teaspoon dried herbs (such as dill or parsley)

Salt and lemon slices for serving.

Instructions:

Preheat the oven to 375°F (190°C).

Place the fish on a baking sheet and brush with olive oil.

Sprinkle with dried herbs and a pinch of salt.

Bake for 12-15 minutes, until the fish flakes easily with a fork.

Serve with lemon slices.

Low-Fiber Pasta with Olive Oil and Parmesan

Ingredients:

1 cup cooked low-fiber pasta (such as white pasta)

1 tablespoon olive oil

2 tablespoons grated Parmesan cheese

Salt to taste

Instructions:

Cook the pasta according to the package directions and drain.

Toss the pasta with olive oil and grated Parmesan cheese.

Season with salt to taste and serve warm.

Egg Salad on White Bread

Ingredients:

2 hard-boiled eggs, chopped.

2 tablespoons mayonnaise

Salt and pepper to taste

2 slices white bread, crusts removed.

Instructions:

In a bowl, mix the chopped eggs with mayonnaise, salt, and pepper.

Spread the egg salad on one slice of white bread, top with the second slice, and cut in half.

Mashed Potato Bowls

Ingredients:

1 cup mashed potatoes

1/2 cup cooked, shredded chicken or turkey

1/4 cup low-sodium gravy

Instructions:

Prepare mashed potatoes without added skins.

Warm the shredded chicken or turkey and the gravy in separate saucepans.

Layer the mashed potatoes at the bottom of a bowl, add the shredded meat, and top with warm gravy.

Baked Apple with Cinnamon

Ingredients:

1 apple cored and sliced.

1/2 teaspoon cinnamon

1 teaspoon sugar (optional)

Instructions:

Preheat the oven to 350°F (175°C).

Place the sliced apple on a baking dish, sprinkle with cinnamon and sugar.

Bake for 20-25 minutes until soft.

Turkey and Cheese Wrap

Ingredients:

1 large, low-fiber tortilla wrap

4 slices turkey breast

2 slices mild cheese (like mozzarella)

Lettuce leaves (optional, if tolerated)

Instructions:

Lay out the tortilla wrap and layer the turkey slices and cheese in the center.

Add lettuce if tolerated.

Roll the tortilla tightly, then cut in half.

Carrot and Ginger Puree

Ingredients:

1 cup peeled and chopped carrots.

1 teaspoon grated ginger

1 cup vegetable broth

Salt to taste

Instructions:

In a saucepan, combine carrots, ginger, and vegetable broth.
Bring to a boil, then reduce heat and simmer until carrots are very soft.

Puree the mixture with a blender until smooth. Season with salt.

Chicken Noodle Soup

Ingredients:

2 cups low-sodium chicken broth

1/2 cup cooked, chopped chicken breast

1/2 cup cooked low-fiber noodles

Salt and pepper to taste

Instructions:

In a pot, bring the chicken broth to a simmer.

Add the cooked chicken and noodles to the broth.

Season with salt and pepper to taste and simmer for a few minutes until heated through.

Creamy Potato Soup

Ingredients:

2 cups peeled and diced potatoes.

1 cup low-sodium vegetable broth

1/2 cup milk

Salt and pepper to taste

Instructions:

In a saucepan, combine the potatoes and vegetable broth.

Bring to a boil, then simmer until the potatoes are tender.

Mash the potatoes in the broth (or blend for a smoother texture).

Stir in the milk and heat through.

Season with salt and pepper.

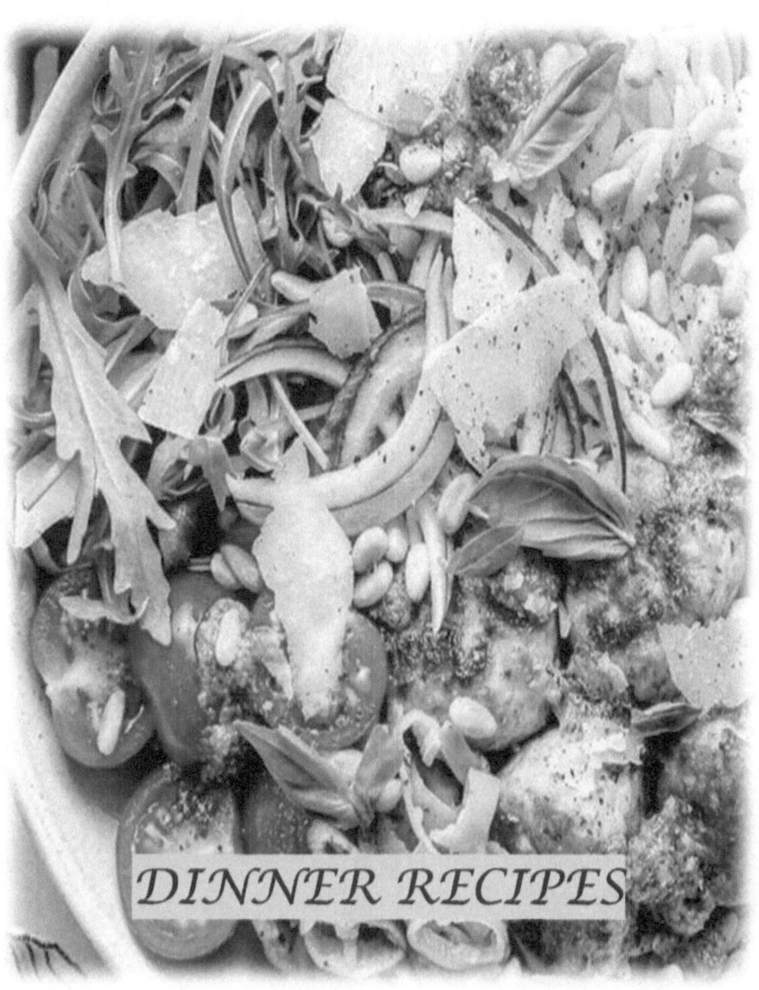

DINNER RECIPES

For individuals managing diverticulitis, choosing dinner recipes that are gentle on the digestive tract is essential, especially during periods of inflammation or recovery. These dinner recipes are designed to be low in fiber and easy on the digestive system, avoiding high-fiber ingredients and focusing on providing nutritious, comforting meals suitable for a diverticulitis-friendly diet.

DINNER RECIPES

Baked Salmon with Lemon

Ingredients:

2 salmon fillets

2 tablespoons olive oil

1 lemon, sliced

Salt and pepper to taste

Instructions:

Preheat the oven to 375°F (190°C).

Arrange the salmon fillets on a baking pan lined with parchment paper.

Drizzle olive oil over the salmon and season with salt and pepper.

Top each fillet with lemon slices.

Bake for 12-15 minutes, or until the salmon is thoroughly cooked and readily flaked with a fork.

Chicken and Zucchini Skillet

Ingredients:

2 boneless, skinless chicken breasts, cut into bite-sized pieces.

1 tablespoon olive oil

2 small zucchinis, peeled and sliced

Salt and pepper to taste

1/2 teaspoon dried oregano

Instructions:

Heat olive oil in a large skillet over moderate heat.

Add the chicken pieces to the skillet and season with salt, pepper, and oregano.

Cook until golden brown and cooked through.

Add the sliced zucchini to the skillet and cook for an additional 5-7 minutes, until the zucchini is tender.

Adjust seasoning if necessary and serve warm.

Tender Beef Stew

Ingredients:

1 pound beef stew meat, cut into small chunks.

2 tablespoons olive oil

2 cups low-sodium beef broth

1 cup peeled and diced potatoes

1 cup peeled and diced carrots

Salt and pepper to taste

Instructions:

In a large pot, heat olive oil over moderate-high heat.

Add the beef chunks and brown on all sides.

Pour in the beef broth and bring to a simmer.

Add the diced potatoes and carrots, then cover and simmer on low heat for 1-1.5 hours, until the beef is tender and the vegetables are cooked.

Season with salt and pepper to taste before serving.

Simple Baked Chicken Breast

Ingredients:

2 boneless, skinless chicken breasts

1 tablespoon olive oil

Salt and pepper to taste

1/2 teaspoon garlic powder (optional)

Instructions:

Preheat the oven to 375°F (190°C).

Rub each chicken breast with olive oil and season with salt, pepper, and garlic powder.

Place the chicken in a baking dish and bake for 20-25 minutes, or until the chicken is cooked through and no longer pink in the center.

Allow the chicken to rest for a few minutes before slicing and serving.

Soft-Cooked Vegetable Puree

Ingredients:

2 cups mixed vegetables (carrots, zucchini, and squash) peeled and diced.

2 tablespoons butter

Salt to taste

Instructions:

Steam the vegetables until very tender.

Transfer the vegetables to a blender, add butter and salt, and puree until smooth.

Adjust the seasoning if needed and serve warm as a side dish or a light dinner option.

Oven-Poached White Fish

Ingredients:

2 white fish fillets (such as cod or tilapia)

1/4 cup low-sodium vegetable broth

1 tablespoon lemon juice

Salt and pepper to taste

Fresh herbs for garnish (optional)

Instructions:

Preheat the oven to 350°F (175°C).

Place each fish fillet on a piece of aluminum foil.

Top with vegetable broth, lemon juice, salt, and pepper.

Fold the foil around the fish, sealing the edges to create a packet.

Bake for 15-20 minutes, until the fish is cooked through.

Garnish with fresh herbs if desired and serve.

Turkey Meatballs in Tomato Sauce

Ingredients:

1 pound ground turkey

1 egg, beaten

2 tablespoons olive oil

1 cup low-sodium tomato sauce

Salt and pepper to taste

Instructions:

In a bowl, mix the ground turkey with the beaten egg, salt, and pepper.

Form into small meatballs.

Heat olive oil in a skillet over medium heat and brown the meatballs on all sides.

Pour the tomato sauce over the meatballs, cover, and simmer for 20 minutes, until the meatballs are cooked through.

Roasted Turkey Breast

Ingredients:

1 turkey breast

2 tablespoons olive oil

Salt and pepper to taste

1 teaspoon dried thyme

Instructions:

Preheat the oven to 350°F (175°C).

Rub the turkey breast with olive oil and season with salt, pepper, and thyme.

Roast in the oven for 60-70 minutes, or until the turkey is cooked through and the internal temperature reaches 165°F (74°C).

Let the turkey rest before slicing.

Soft Baked Cod with Parsley

Ingredients:

2 cod fillets

1 tablespoon olive oil

Salt and pepper to taste

1 tablespoon chopped fresh parsley.

Instructions:

Preheat the oven to 375°F (190°C).

Place cod fillets in a baking dish and drizzle with olive oil.

Season with salt and pepper.

Bake for 12-15 minutes, until the fish is opaque and flakes easily.

Sprinkle with fresh parsley before serving.

Carrot Soup

Ingredients:

2 cups peeled and chopped carrots.

4 cups low-sodium vegetable broth

1 onion, chopped

2 tablespoons olive oil

Salt and pepper to taste

Instructions:

In a large pot, heat the olive oil over medium heat.

Add the onion and cook until translucent.

Add the carrots and cook for a few minutes, then add the vegetable broth.

Bring to a boil, then simmer until the carrots are very soft, about 20 minutes.

Puree the soup with an immersion blender or in batches using a regular blender until smooth.

Return the soup to the pot, reheat gently, and season with salt and pepper to taste.

Serve warm, optionally garnished with a swirl of cream or a sprinkle of fresh herbs for added flavor.

SOUP RECIPES

When managing diverticulitis, especially during flare-ups, it's crucial to consume foods that minimize irritation to the digestive tract. Soups can be an excellent option as they're easy to digest and can be packed with nutrients. Here are soup recipes designed with a diverticulitis diet in mind, focusing on low-fiber and easily digestible ingredients.

SOUP RECIPES

Chicken Broth Soup

Ingredients:

4 cups low-sodium chicken broth

1 cup cooked, shredded chicken

Salt and pepper to taste

Instructions:

In a large pot, bring the chicken broth to a simmer.

Season the saucepan with salt and pepper before adding the shredded chicken.

Let Simmer for 10 minutes. Serve warm.

Simple Beef Broth

Ingredients:

4 cups low-sodium beef broth

1 cup cooked, diced lean beef.

Salt and pepper to taste

Instructions:

In a large pot, bring the beef broth to a simmer.

Add the cooked beef and season with salt and pepper.

Let it simmer for 10 minutes to allow the flavors to meld.

Serve warm.

Carrot and Potato Soup

Ingredients:

2 cups peeled and diced carrots.

2 cups peeled and diced potatoes

4 cups low-sodium vegetable broth

Salt to taste

1 tablespoon olive oil

Instructions:

In a large pot, heat the olive oil over moderate heat.

Add the carrots and potatoes, cooking until slightly softened, about 5 minutes.

Add the vegetable broth and bring to a boil.

Reduce heat and simmer until the vegetables are tender, about 20 minutes.

Puree the soup using an immersion blender until smooth. Season with salt. Serve warm.

Butternut Squash Soup

Ingredients:

2 cups peeled and cubed butternut squash.

3 cups low-sodium chicken or vegetable broth

Salt to taste

1 tablespoon olive oil

¼ cup milk (optional, for creaminess)

Instructions:

In a large pot, heat the olive oil over moderate heat.

Add the butternut squash and cook for a few minutes until it starts to soften.

Add the broth and bring to a boil.

Reduce heat and simmer until the squash is completely tender, about 25 minutes.

Puree the soup until smooth.

Stir in milk if using, for added creaminess.

Season with salt. Serve warm.

Gentle Lentil Soup

Ingredients:

1 cup red lentils rinsed and drained.

4 cups low-sodium vegetable broth

Salt to taste

1 tablespoon olive oil

1/2 teaspoon ground turmeric (optional, for its anti-inflammatory properties)

Instructions:

In a large pot, heat the olive oil over moderate heat.

Add the turmeric and whisk for about 30 seconds.

Add the red lentils and vegetable broth.

Bring to a boil, then simmer until the lentils are soft, about 15 minutes.

Puree half the soup for a smoother texture with some lentil bits remaining.

Season with salt. Serve warm.

Creamy Potato Leek Soup

Ingredients:

2 cups peeled and diced potatoes.

1 cup sliced leeks (white part only)

3 cups low-sodium chicken or vegetable broth

Salt to taste

1 tablespoon butter

Instructions:

In a large pot, melt the butter over moderate heat.

Cook the leeks until tender, about 5 minutes.

Add the potatoes and broth.

Bring to a boil, then reduce heat and simmer for 20

minutes, or until the potatoes are cooked.

Puree the soup until smooth.

Season with salt.

Serve warm.

Tomato Basil Soup

Ingredients:

4 cups canned, no-salt-added, peeled tomatoes (blended)

2 tablespoons fresh basil, chopped

2 cups low-sodium vegetable broth

Salt to taste

1 tablespoon olive oil

Instructions:

In a large pot, heat the olive oil over moderate heat.

Add the blended tomatoes and vegetable broth.

Bring to a simmer and cook for 20 minutes.

Add the chopped basil and season with salt.

Simmer for an additional 5 minutes.

Serve warm.

Zucchini Soup

Ingredients:

2 cups peeled and sliced zucchini.

3 cups low-sodium chicken or vegetable broth

Salt to taste

1 tablespoon olive oil

Instructions:

In a large pot, heat the olive oil over moderate heat.

Add the zucchini and cook until soft, about 10 minutes.

Add the broth and bring to a boil.

Reduce heat and simmer for 15 minutes.

Puree the soup until smooth.

Season with salt.

Serve warm.

Acorn Squash Soup

Ingredients:

2 cups peeled and cubed acorn squash.

3 cups low-sodium chicken or vegetable broth

Salt to taste

1 tablespoon olive oil

¼ teaspoon ground nutmeg (optional, for flavor)

Instructions:

In a large pot, heat the olive oil over moderate heat.

Add the acorn squash and cook until it begins to soften, about 5 minutes.

Add the broth and bring to a boil.

Reduce the heat to low and simmer until the squash is completely tender, about 25 minutes.

Add the ground nutmeg if using, for a hint of warmth and depth.

Puree the soup with an immersion blender until smooth. If you don't have an immersion blender, let the soup cool slightly before pureeing it in batches in a regular blender.

Season with salt to taste. Serve warm, garnished with a sprinkle of nutmeg or a few fresh herbs if desired.

Parsnip and Apple Soup

Ingredients:

2 cups peeled and chopped parsnips.

1 cup peeled and diced apple (sweet varieties work best)

3 cups low-sodium chicken or vegetable broth

Salt to taste

1 tablespoon olive oil

A pinch of cinnamon (optional, for a sweet and savory flavor profile)

Instructions:

In a large pot, heat the olive oil over moderate heat.

Add the parsnips and apple, cooking until they start to soften, about 10 minutes.

Add the broth and bring the mixture to a boil.

Reduce the heat and simmer until the parsnips and apples are very tender, about 20 minutes.

Stir in a pinch of cinnamon if using, to enhance the soup's flavor.

Puree the soup until smooth, either using an immersion blender directly in the pot or by transferring the soup in batches to a blender. Be cautious if using a blender with hot liquids.

Season with salt to taste. Serve warm, enjoying the unique blend of parsnips' earthiness with the gentle sweetness of apples.

Each of these soup recipes is crafted to be gentle on the digestive system, making them suitable for those managing diverticulitis, especially during times of inflammation. Remember, individual tolerances to certain foods can vary, so it's important to listen to your body and adjust ingredients as needed.

SNACKS RECIPES

Creating snacks suitable for a diverticulitis diet, especially during flare-ups, means focusing on low-fiber and easily digestible foods. Here are snack recipes designed to be gentle on the digestive system while providing nourishment and satisfaction.

Baked Apple Chips

Ingredients:

2 apples (choose a sweet variety)

A sprinkle of cinnamon (optional)

Instructions:

Preheat your oven to 200°F (93°C).

Core the apples and slice them very thinly.

Arrange the apple slices on a baking sheet coated with parchment paper.

If desired, sprinkle lightly with cinnamon.

Bake for 1-2 hours, flipping halfway through, until the apple slices are dried out but still pliable.

Allow it to cool before serving.

Smooth Peanut Butter Banana Smoothie

Ingredients:

1 ripe banana
2 tablespoons smooth peanut butter
1 cup almond milk or other non-dairy milk
Ice cubes (optional)

Instructions:

Combine the banana, peanut butter, and almond milk in a blender.

Add ice cubes if you prefer a colder smoothie.

Blend until smooth. Serve immediately.

Mashed Avocado on Rice Cakes

Ingredients:

1 ripe avocado

Salt and lemon juice to taste

Rice cakes

Instructions:

In a bowl, mash the avocado with a fork until smooth.

Season with a little salt and lemon juice to taste.

Spread the mashed avocado evenly on rice cakes.

Serve immediately.

Baked Sweet Potato Fries

Ingredients:

2 sweet potatoes, peeled.

1 tablespoon olive oil

Salt to taste

Instructions:

Preheat your oven to 400°F (200°C).

Cut the sweet potatoes into thin fries.

Toss the fries with olive oil and salt.

Spread the fries on a baking sheet in a single layer.

Bake for 20-25 minutes, turning once, until they are golden and crisp. Serve warm.

Homemade Banana Pudding

Ingredients:

2 ripe bananas

2 cups almond milk

2 tablespoons honey

2 tablespoons cornstarch

Instructions:

In a blender, combine bananas, almond milk, and honey. Blend until smooth.

Pour the mixture into a saucepan.

Whisk in the cornstarch.

Cook over moderate heat, stirring constantly, until the mixture thickens.

Pour into bowls and refrigerate until set.

Serve chilled.

Cucumber and Hummus Cups

Ingredients:

1 large cucumber

½ cup hummus

Instructions:

Slice the cucumber into thick rounds.

Using a small spoon, scoop out the center of each cucumber round to create a small cup.

Fill each cucumber cup with hummus.

Serve immediately.

Cottage Cheese and Pineapple

Ingredients:

1 cup low-fat cottage cheese

½ cup diced pineapple (fresh or canned in juice)

Instructions:

Combine the cottage cheese and pineapple in a bowl.

Serve chilled.

Soft Baked Pears

Ingredients:

2 pears halved and cored.

A sprinkle of cinnamon (optional)

A drizzle of honey (optional)

Instructions:

Preheat your oven to 350°F (175°C).

Place the pear halves on a baking sheet, cut sides up.

If desired, sprinkle with cinnamon and drizzle with honey.

Bake for 20-25 minutes or until the pears are soft.

Serve warm.

Avocado Chocolate Mousse

Ingredients:

1 ripe avocado

2 tablespoons cocoa powder

2 tablespoons honey or maple syrup

½ teaspoon vanilla extract

Almond milk, as needed for consistency.

Instructions:

In a blender, combine the avocado, cocoa powder, honey/maple syrup, and vanilla extract.

Blend until smooth, adding a little almond milk as needed to achieve a mousse-like consistency.

Refrigerate until chilled.

Serve cold.

Yogurt with Honey and Almonds

Ingredients:

1 cup low-fat Greek yogurt

2 tablespoons honey

A handful of sliced almonds

Instructions:

Spoon the Greek yogurt into a bowl.

Drizzle with honey and sprinkle with sliced almonds.

Serve immediately.

CONCLUSION

"EASY TO PREPARE DIVERTICULITIS DIET COOKBOOK" it's essential to reflect on the journey this book has undertaken to guide those affected by diverticulitis through a dietary path that is both healing and nourishing. Through careful selection of ingredients and crafting of recipes, this cookbook aims to provide not only relief during flare-ups but also a foundation for long-term dietary habits that support digestive health.

The recipes within these pages, from soothing breakfasts to comforting dinners and gentle snacks, have been designed with the utmost consideration for the delicate balance required in a diverticulitis-friendly diet. Each dish is crafted to minimize digestive stress while maximizing nutritional value, ensuring that individuals can enjoy a wide range of flavors and textures without compromising their health.

In closing, may this cookbook inspire you to explore new flavors, to cherish the act of cooking as a form of self-care, and to enjoy the journey towards a balanced, healthy digestive system.

Here's to finding peace in every meal and strength in every bite.

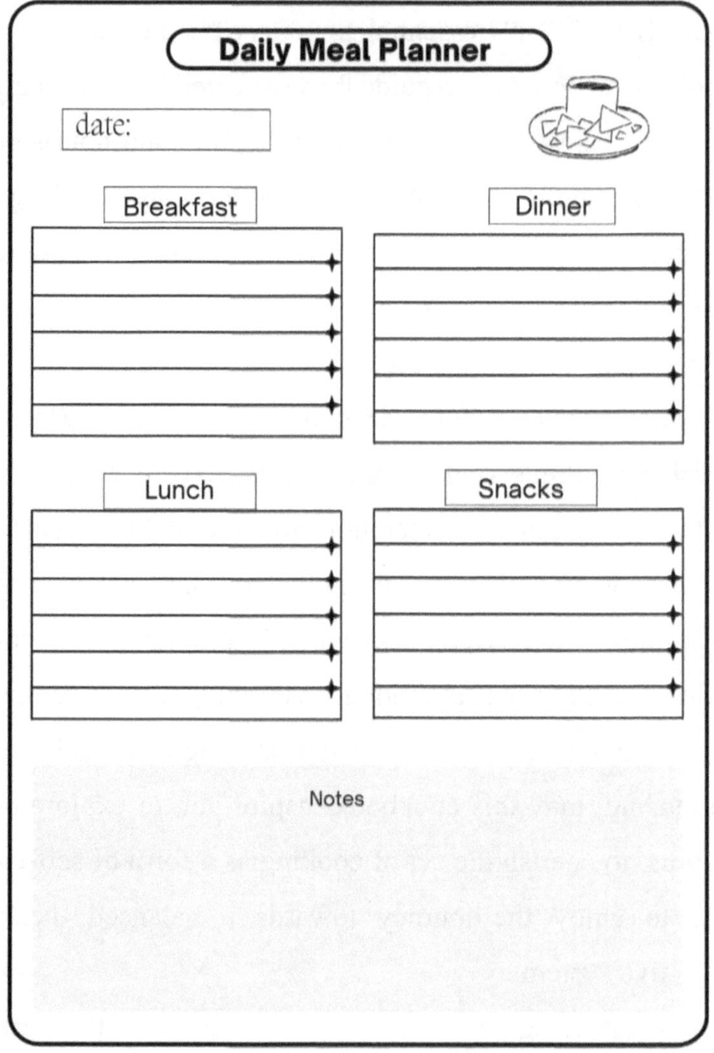

Daily Meal Planner
date:
Breakfast
Dinner
Lunch
Snacks
Notes

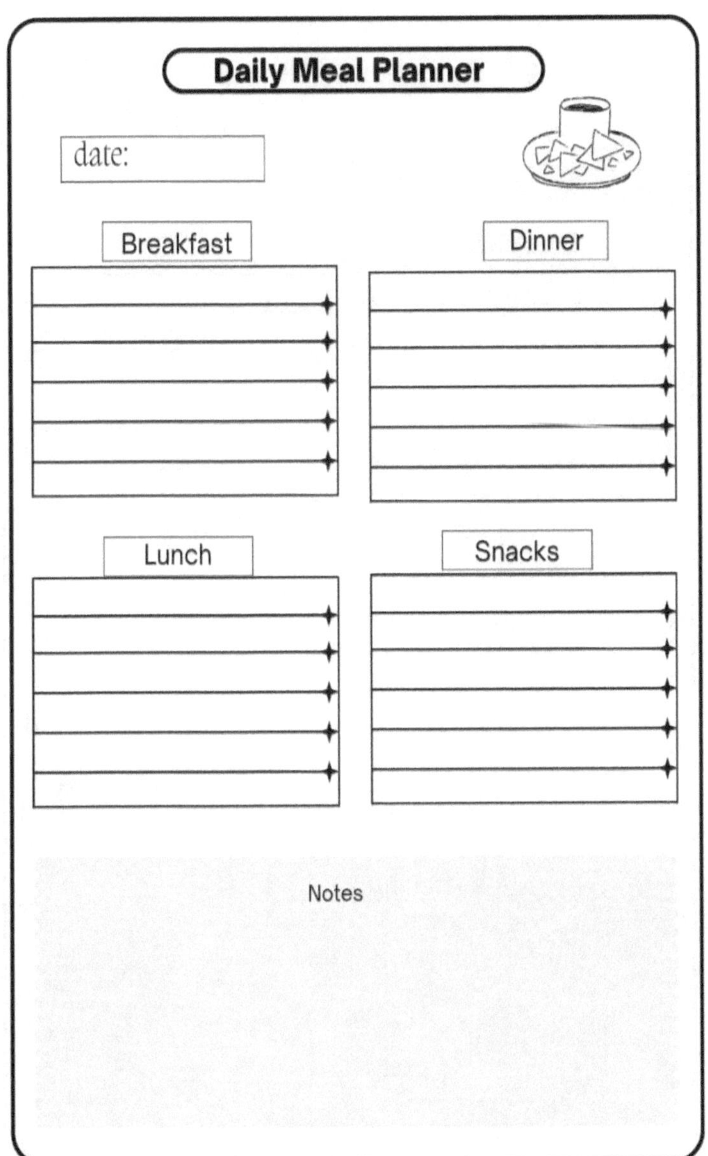

Daily Meal Planner
date:
Breakfast
Dinner
Lunch
Snacks
Notes

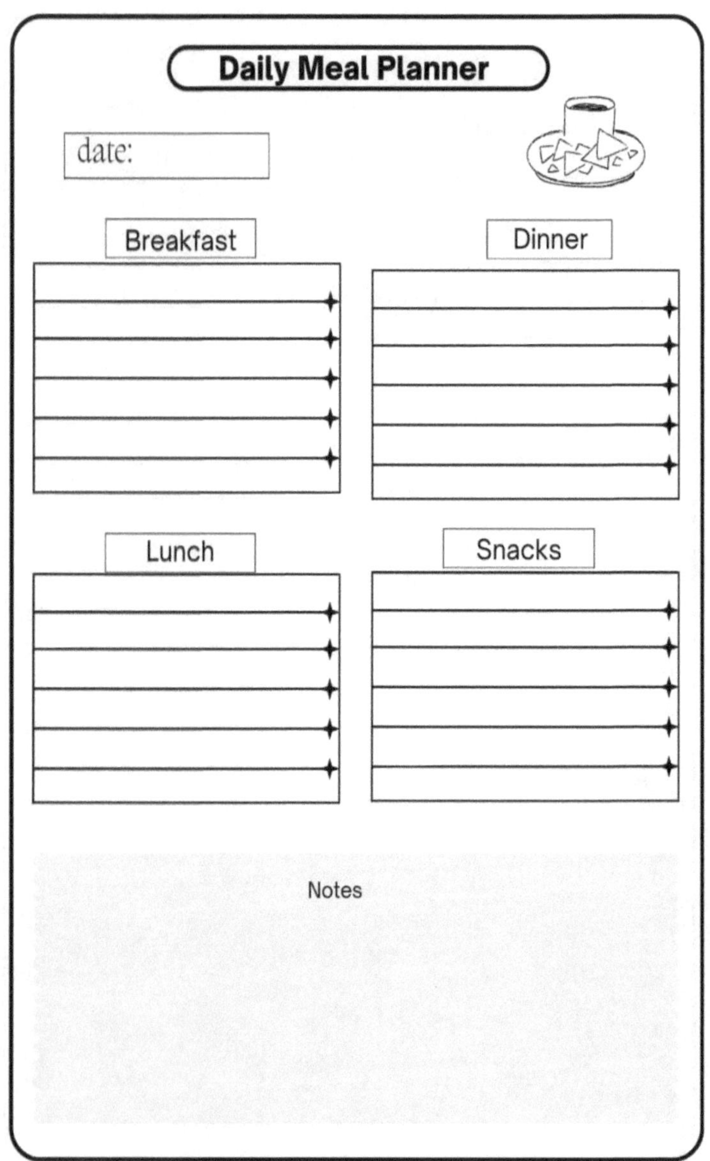

Daily Meal Planner
date:
Breakfast
Dinner
Lunch
Snacks
Notes

Daily Meal Planner

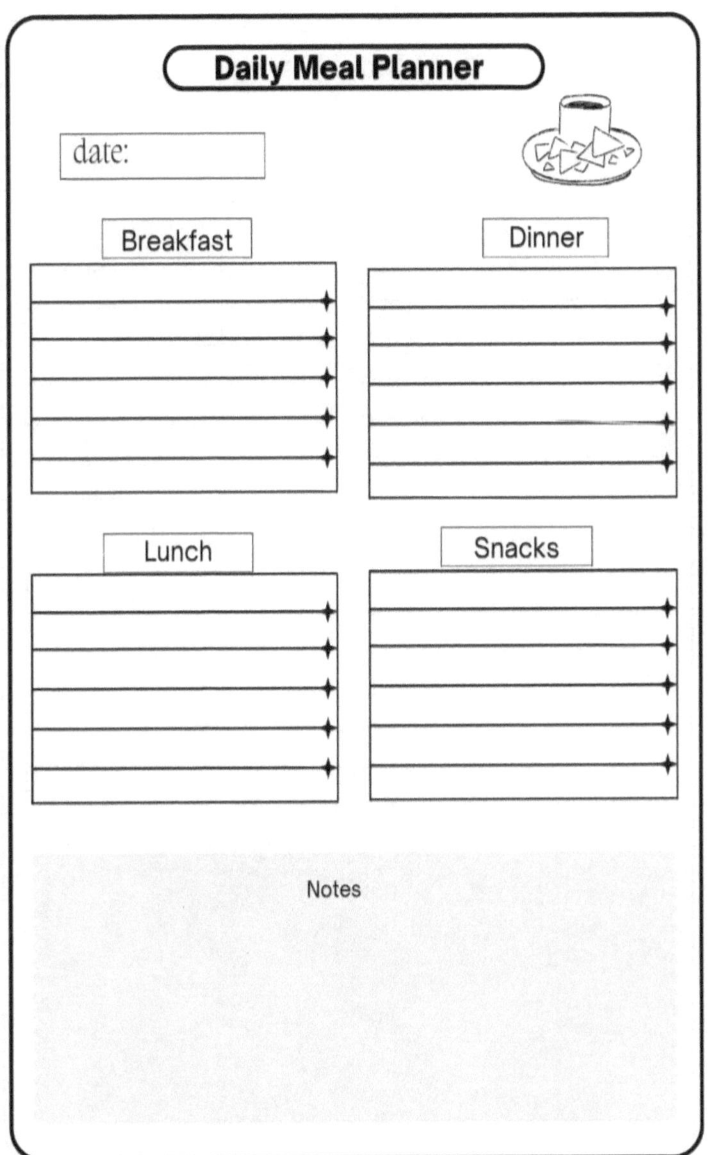

date:

Breakfast

Dinner

Lunch

Snacks

Notes

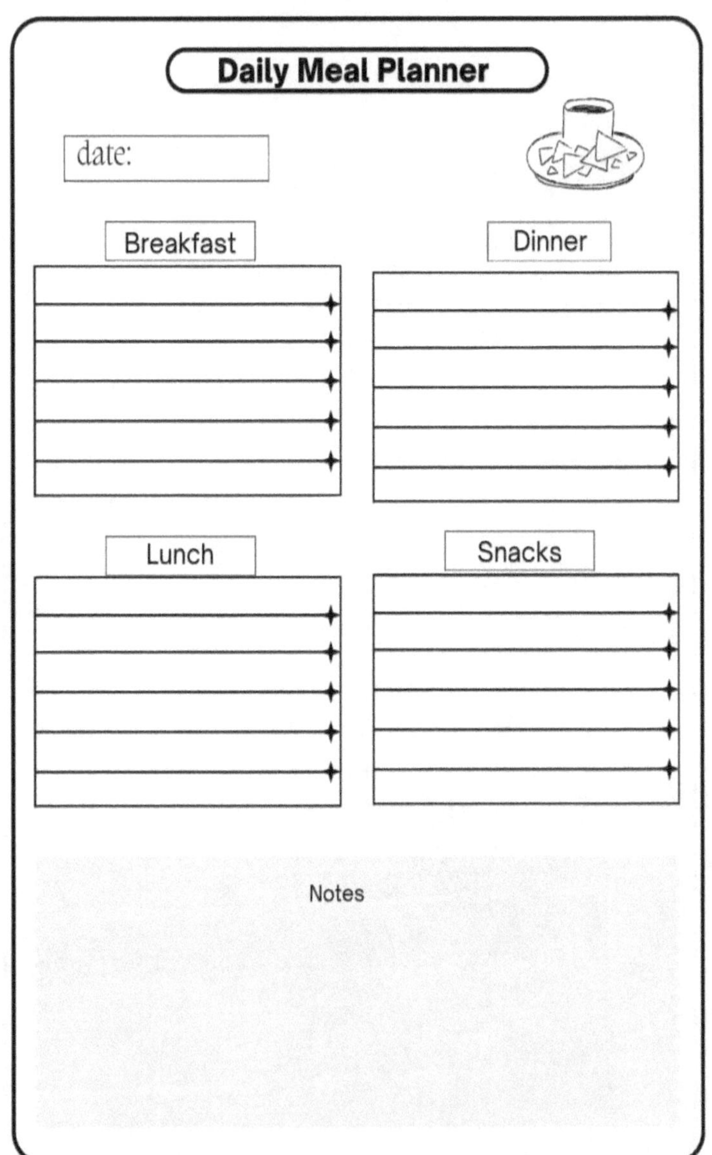

Daily Meal Planner

date:

Breakfast

Dinner

Lunch

Snacks

Notes

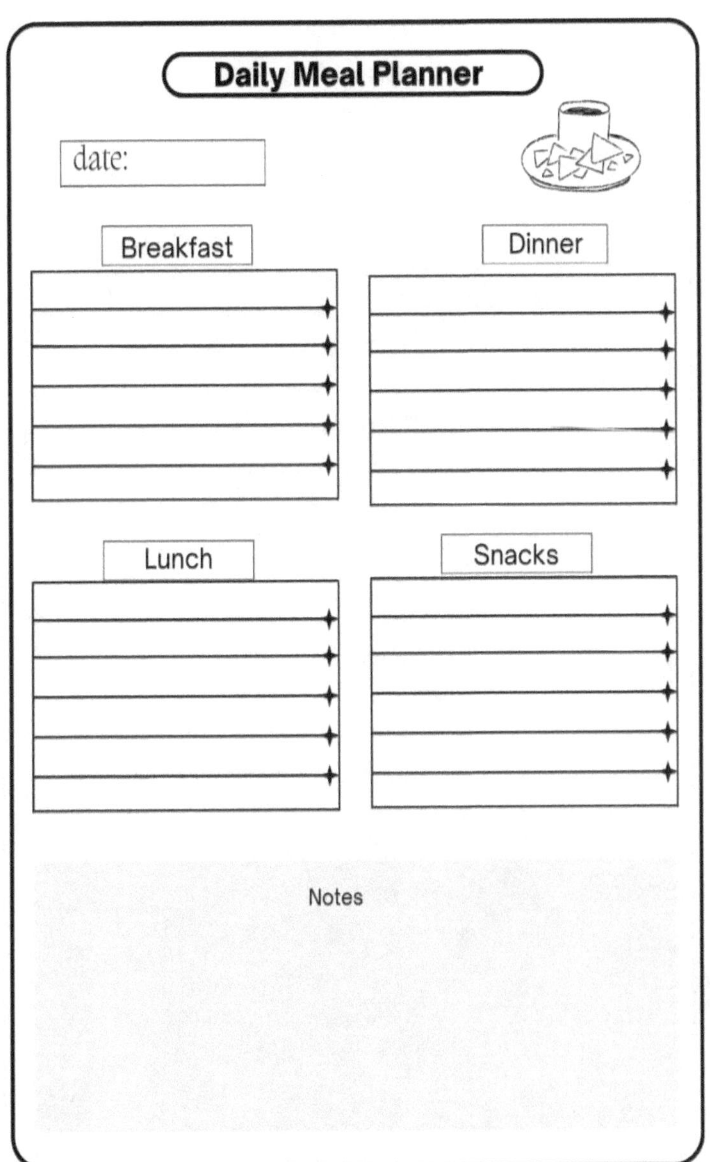

Daily Meal Planner
date:
Breakfast
Dinner
Lunch
Snacks
Notes

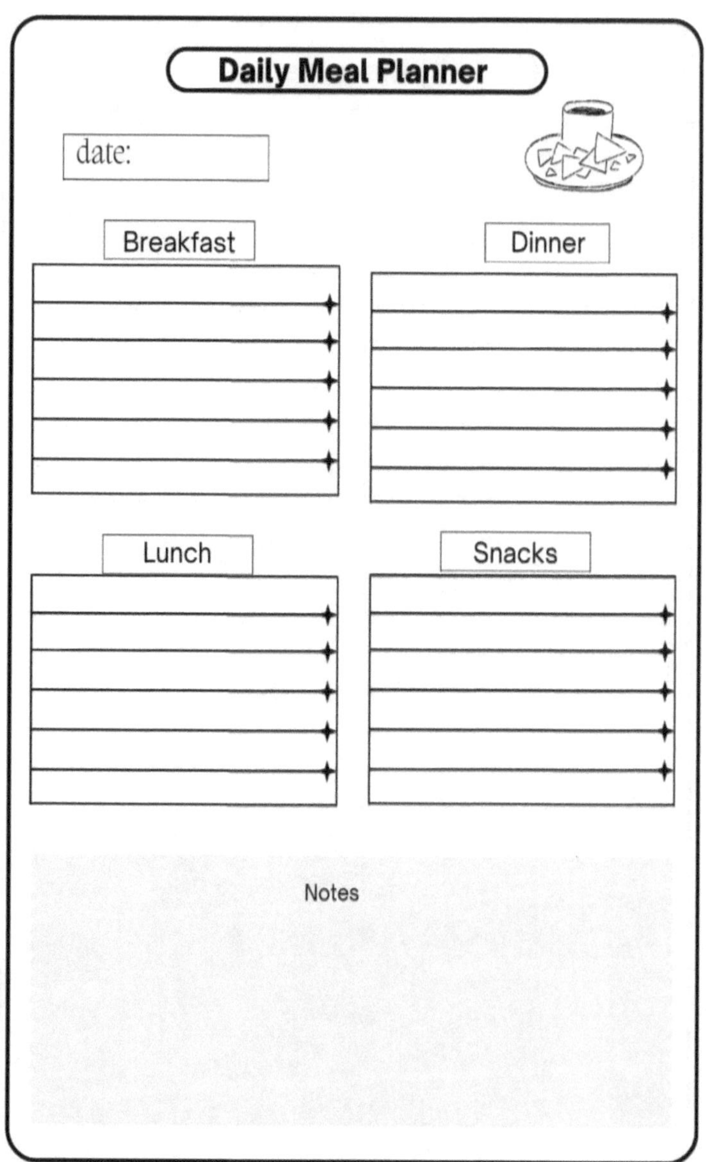
Daily Meal Planner
date:
Breakfast
Dinner
Lunch
Snacks
Notes

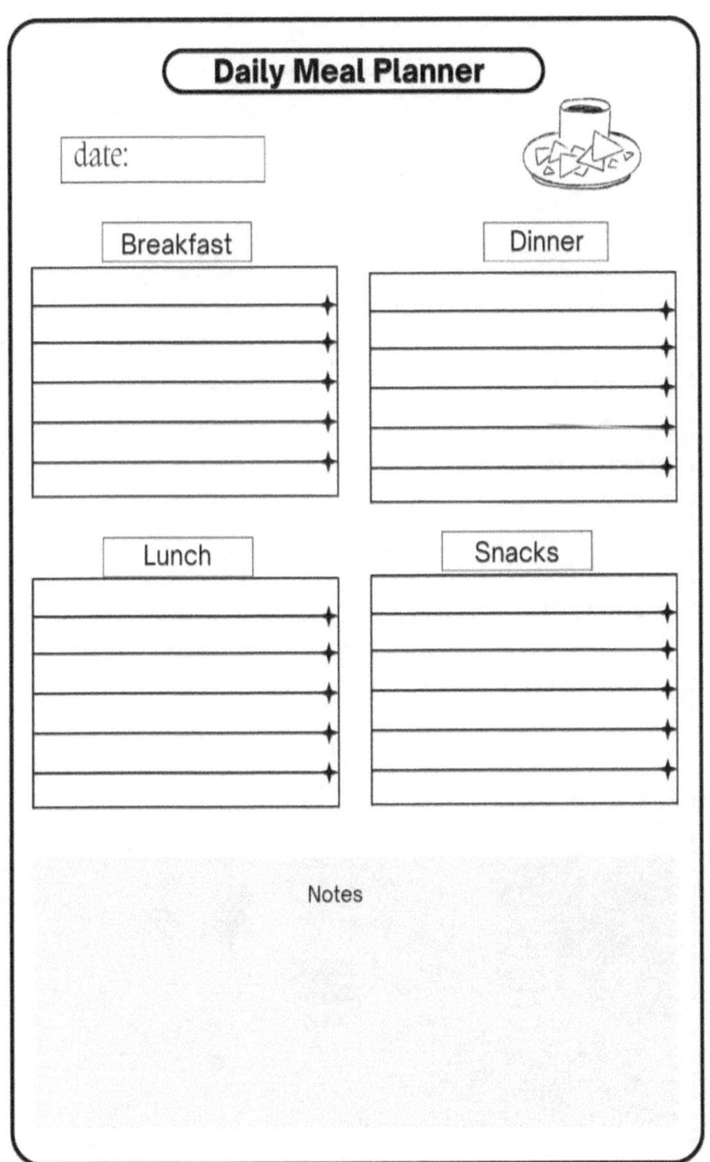

Daily Meal Planner
date:
Breakfast
Dinner
Lunch
Snacks
Notes

Daily Meal Planner

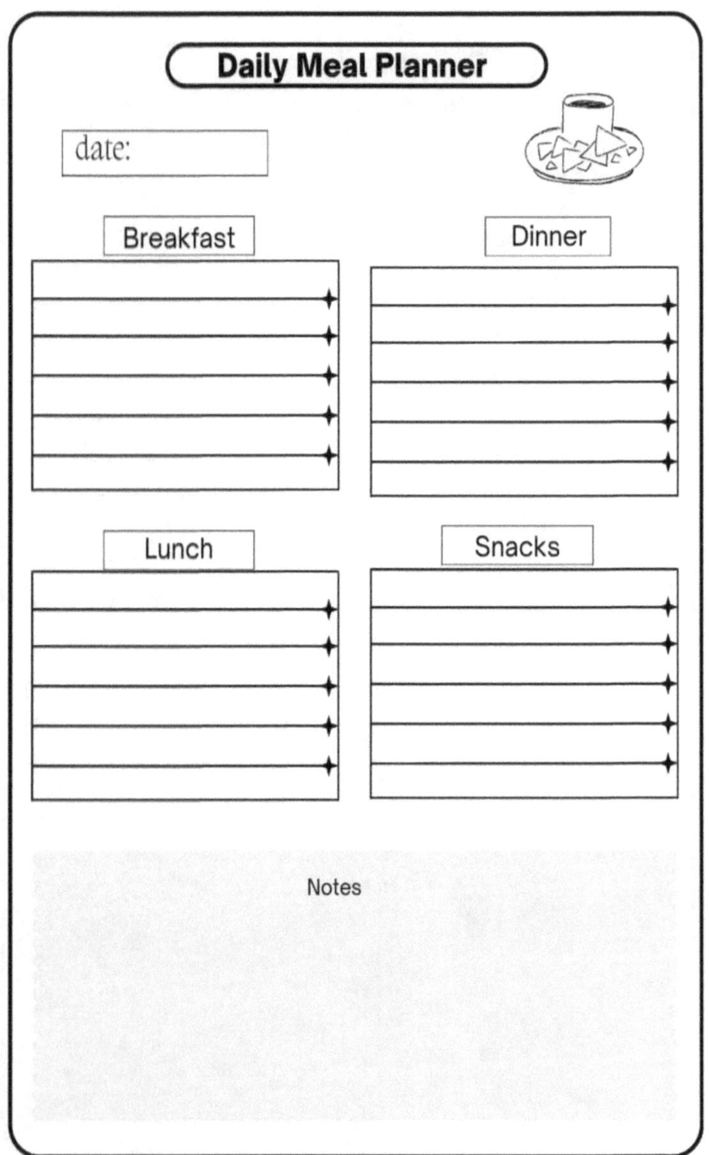

date:

Breakfast

Dinner

Lunch

Snacks

Notes

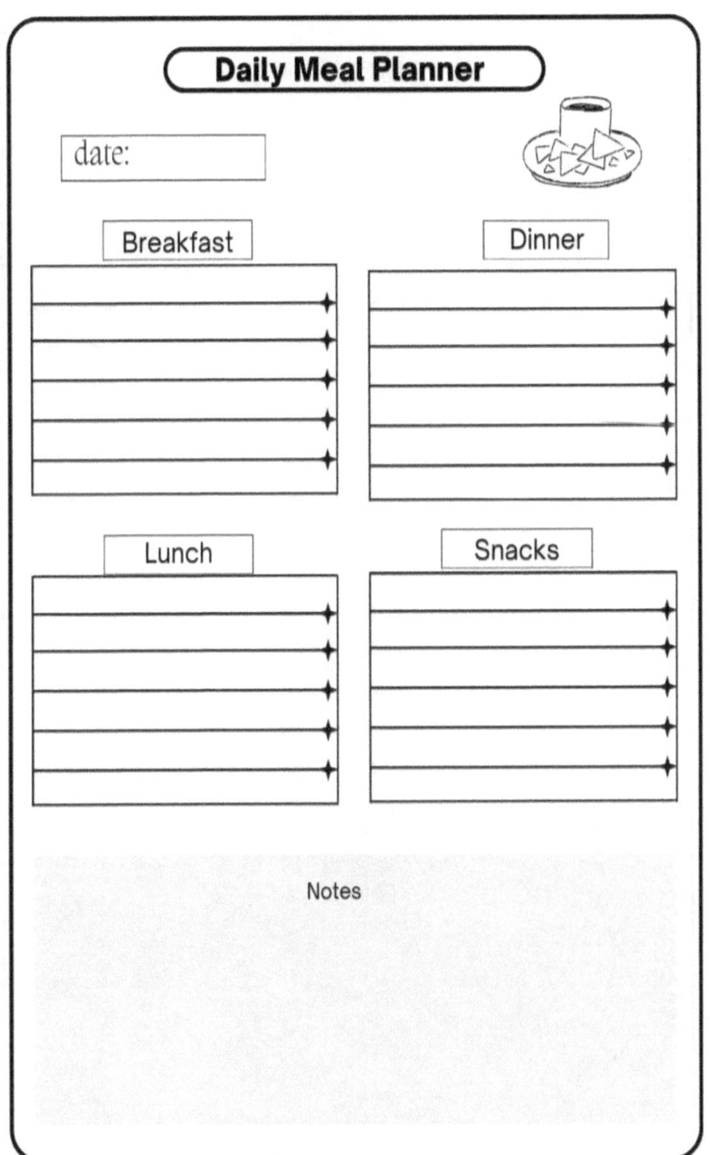

Daily Meal Planner

date:

Breakfast

Dinner

Lunch

Snacks

Notes

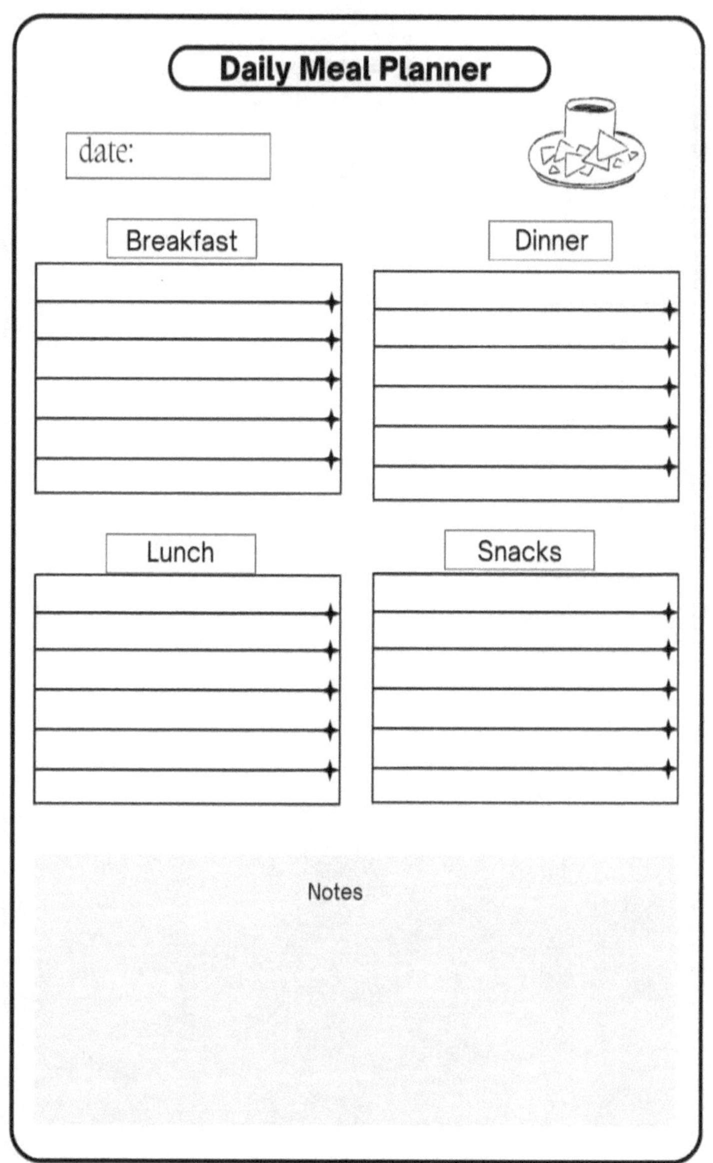

Daily Meal Planner
date:
Breakfast
Dinner
Lunch
Snacks
Notes

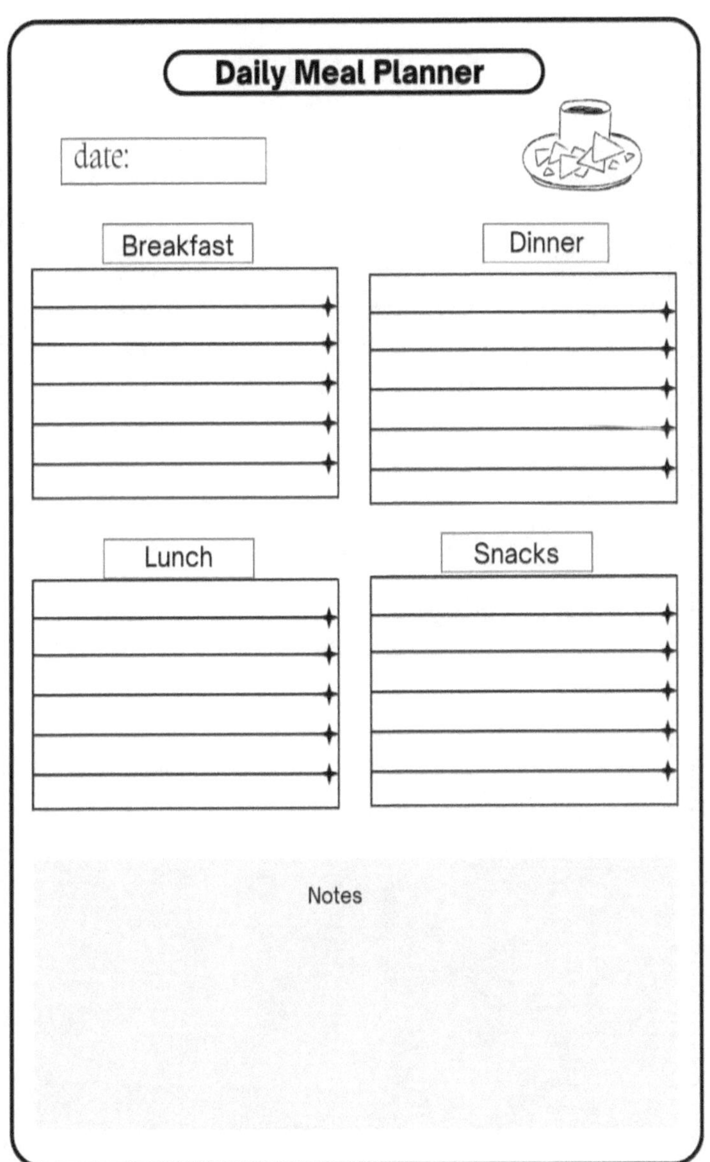

Daily Meal Planner

date:

Breakfast

Dinner

Lunch

Snacks

Notes

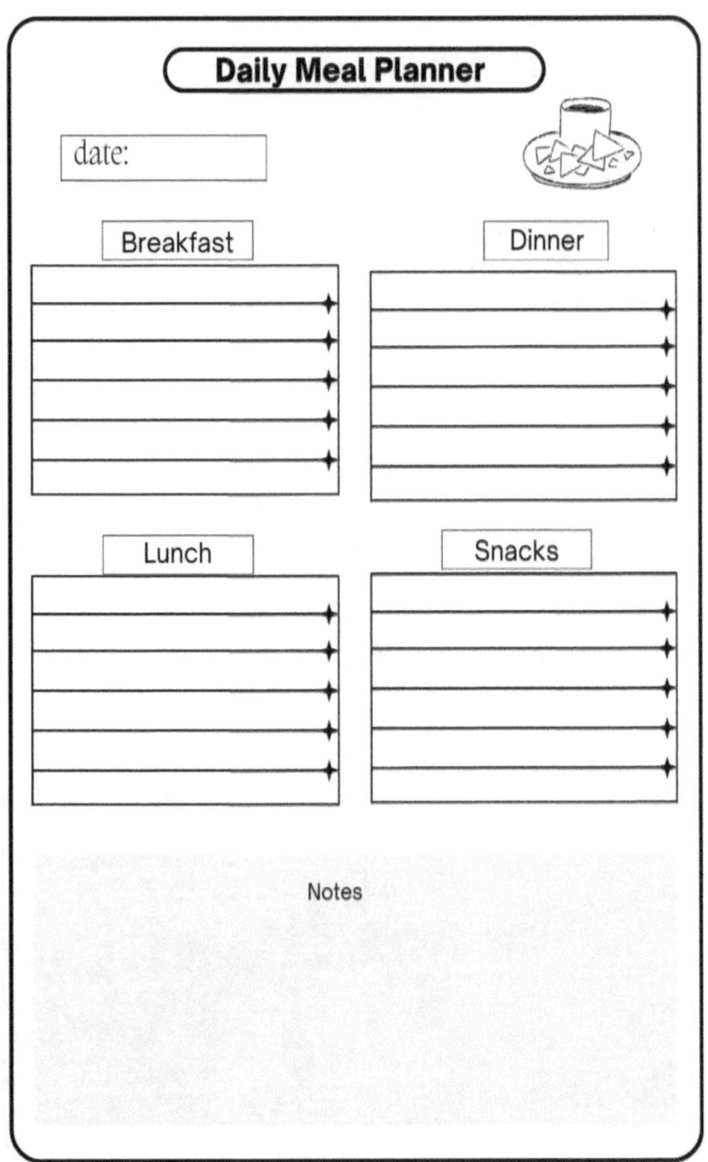

Daily Meal Planner
date:
Breakfast
Dinner
Lunch
Snacks
Notes

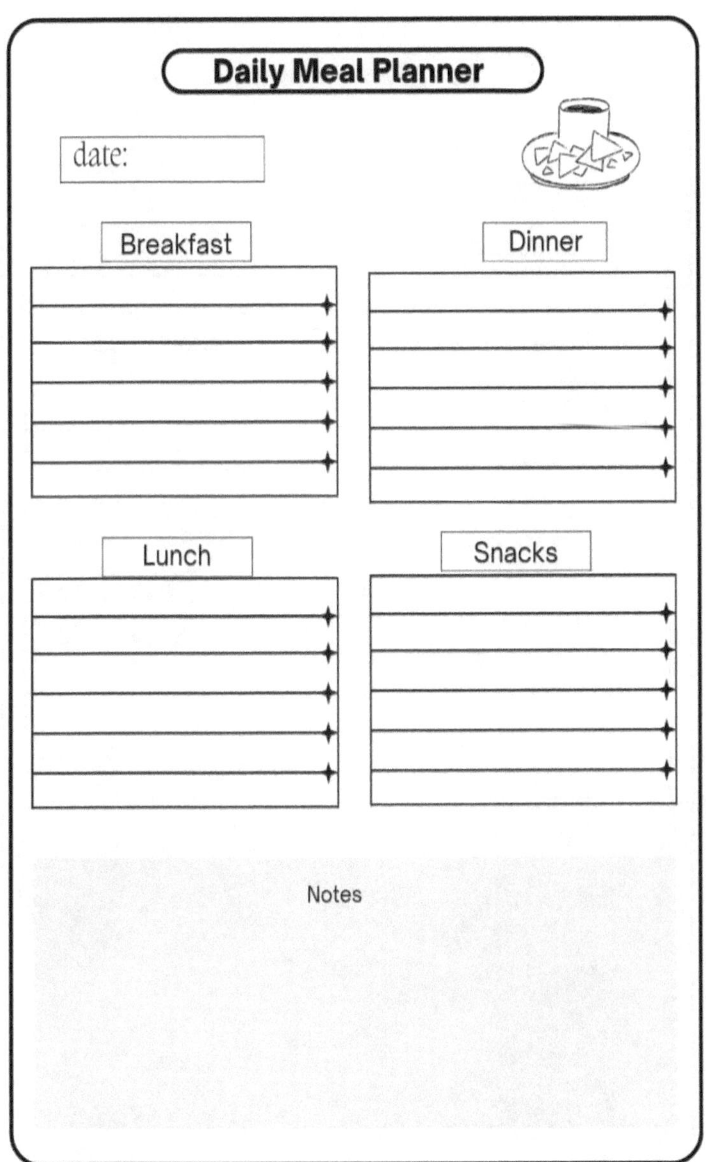

Daily Meal Planner
date:
Breakfast
Dinner
Lunch
Snacks
Notes

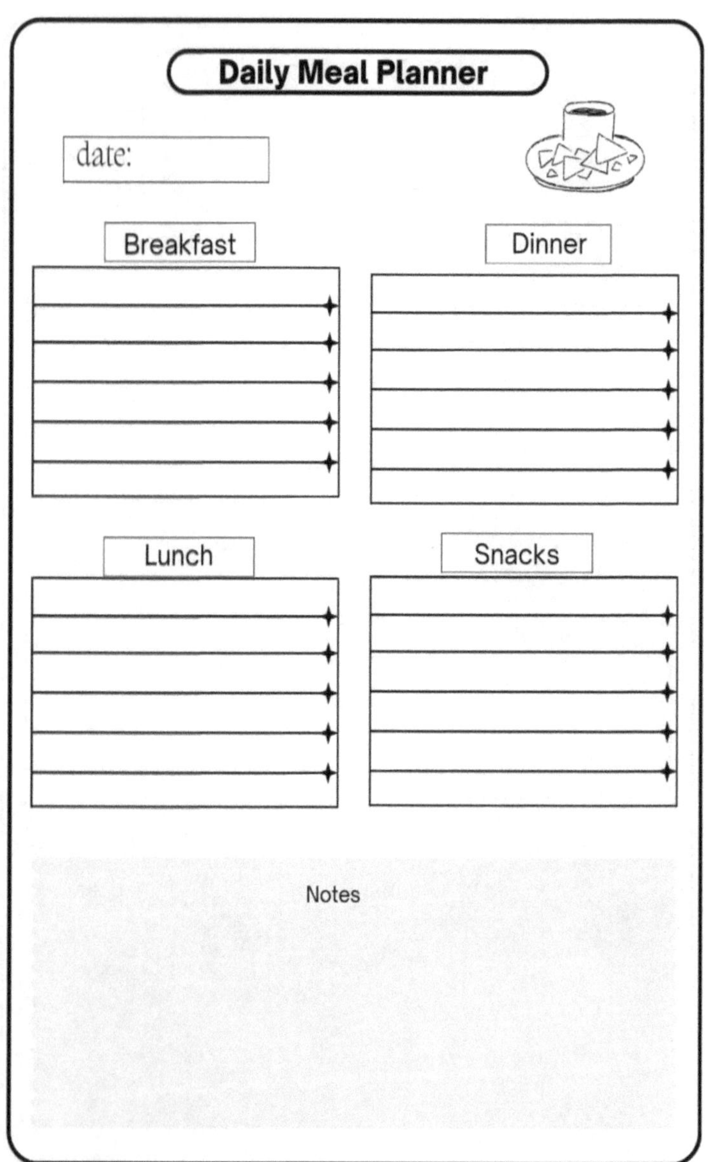

Daily Meal Planner

date:

Breakfast

Dinner

Lunch

Snacks

Notes